Pregnant

&

Empowered

Elizabeth Clyde

The information and other content provided in this **book are** not intended, and should not be construed as **medical** advice, nor is the information a substitute for professional **medical** expertise or treatment.

I desire to see more hospitals work with midwives and doulas to help improve the birthing process across the globe. Hospitals have the budget to help midwives and doulas sustain their careers, and collectively we can work towards a better health outcome for all mothers and children.

Dedication:

To my husband, Jeral Clyde II: You are my rock and strength; I love you beyond words!

Let us keep doing it our way and trusting the process.

Your One True Love Always,

Elizabeth

Contents

Note: Use all additional pages to take notes or simply to journal. <3

Introduction

My goal for this book is not to overwhelm you. Initially, I began with infusing stories of other women into the book, and then I realized it may be better to make this about me and you. Me, a millennial mother that has given birth to both of my children in the comfort of my home. You, in all your glory, potentially being a mother, birth worker, doula, midwife, nurse, doctor, spouse, or simply someone interested in the journey of birth, I welcome you on this journey with me.

I want you to first understand that birth is mental. If you are familiar with working out your physical body this is the time when it is vital to work on your mental strength. Fear has no place in birth, and if you are fearful, it will impact your outcome. If you are presently with-child, have you really sat and embraced the true miracle of life inside of you?

I want to connect you with finding JOY in the JOURNEY.

Please allow me to preface this by saying although I have successfully birthed both of our sons at home, my intention in authoring this book is not about that. I feel that now more than ever it is time for the birthing community to rally around mothers to empower them to bring forth the next generation, someone must do it.

Many people talk about population increase and such, but many of the mother's I know with multiple children believe in legacy, honor, and leaving the world in a better place than it is today. I am not here to convince you of anything. My goal is simply to empower you in your own ability to make the best-informed decision on how to best bring your children into the world.

This book will provide to you, a 3-day journal by trimester (accompanied with common symptoms) along with the birth stories of both son's: Champion-Jeral III and Dominion. I searched high and low for first-time home birth stories or at least a mother that could tell me she even had a positive birth story. I kept running into women who told me how the birth experience robbed them or that they lost a child giving birth.

There is a woman who shared with me that her male doctor used both of his hands and strength to "help" her stretch for the baby. Afterwards, she was stitched up and told that it was normal for the doctor to pull her apart and that he was simply assisting. She shared with me that she was traumatized from that experience and her husband desired more children. However, she could not bring herself to go through birth again. It was nothing I could do or say, just listen to her talk from her soul.

My belief, based on my experience, is that the body was made to stretch when in the proper position. In the home birth community olive oil has been used to assist with slip as well as birthing while standing instead of being on one's back is a method that can be encouraged.

In the capacity I have seen olive oil utilized it is simply drizzled down the middle of the woman's back while she is in an upright position to assist her in multiple ways with the main goal being to prevent tearing. The intimacy of home birth involves complete surrender and a trusted support system.

I have not torn after either birth because the home birth environment encourages movement (standing while leaning over and holding onto something or someone to steady oneself during intense waves is helpful). What If I told you, the energy of birth outcomes being positive or negative can be impacted based on who is present for the experience? You may not be afraid or intimidated by birth, so protect your spirit and be wise in choosing your method and audience for your birth.

I had to forge my own path and stick to my instincts. I later found out that my great-aunt gave birth to her 8 children at home, and she is currently still alive at 101 years of age. Prior to knowing that piece of family history I was simply instinctually determined to push past social norms despite my own fears of the unknown. I kept telling myself that the outcome would be no one's responsibility other than my own whether positive or negative. I had to choose to give myself the best birth experience. There are countless other women that have gone before me, and so I want to be clear: I am no different than you. Allow us now to begin.

With Genuine Love,

Elizabeth

@MrsElClyde5

First Trimester

The symptoms you see below are some that I have experienced, and you may as well. However, it is best not to compare, it may just be **different** for you!

Let us begin with knowing and understanding every woman's birthing journey is unique and tailored to them. I know I have heard so many diverse pregnancy and birth experiences that I truly just desire God to grant us all a graceful healthy journey while we bring forth life into the world. It is a duty and calling for women who choose such a path, and it will bring you great honor.

<u>Symptoms</u>

Food Aversions

Missed Period

Nausea

Fatigue

Irritability

Increased Need to Tinkle (Urinate)

Emotional Sensitivity

Long Naps

Increased Heart Rate

Constipation

Tender Breasts

Uncontrollable Laughter or Tears

I know that there is content out there that gives you information week by week of your pregnancy. What I have found is that sometimes I can worry unnecessarily as I begin to review more information online. I do not know about you, but there are some posts on these birth sites I just do not need to read.

For pregnancy, I recommend protecting your mind more than anything. My strongest recommendation is that a mother focus on her alignment with the Lord her God. You may come from a family that frowns upon bringing forth life and let me be the first to tell you others' opinions of you have nothing to do with the task at hand. The fact of the matter is once conception is made, mother and baby are now the focus.

Focus as much as you can on the excitement of pregnancy and eat to your heart's content because I know rest and food to be essential for pregnant mothers. I personally must have at least a light snack every two-hours, and that is without being pregnant.

The only times I have experienced not holding down my food while pregnant was when I waited too long to eat. I recommend eating at least every two hours if you have an appetite. In my first trimester I take in a lot of fluids as I can be parched during that beginning stage.

My personal strategy with prenatal vitamins is that I take them after birth up until conception. Once I am with-child, I steer towards taking in the needed vitamins through food.

For some reason prenatal vitamins when I am pregnant cause me to feel nauseous and lightheaded. I spoke to my midwife about it and even researched it online that some doctors will even advise a mother to find another way to get the nutrients that prenatal vitamins provide.

As far as constipation goes, I have reasoned with myself that it makes sense for the body to hold onto more nutrients and make it more difficult to expel them to ensure the baby has what is needed within the womb. There will be many things you will experience that are new to you, and at the end of the book I will provide resources that I have used to enable me to birth with a knowledge of what is taking place.

Try doing more research on what your baby is doing in the womb, the developmental process and find the foods that make you feel great.

Note: If you are pregnant and lack the support system that you feel is needed, I petition to you that before you make any decision, I ask that you simply email me: biz@elizabethclyde.com I may be able to assist, and even if I am not that first trimester is filled with a roller coaster of emotions that cannot always be trusted. Emotions and feelings can often change if the right perspective is given. I prefer we exhaust all efforts and see what resources are available. Ok, dear? Ok! Even if you need someone to talk to, there is no judgment, and we can get through it together. Try closing your eyes and taking deep breaths. If a few tears roll down your face during that moment, then you know you are simply releasing what's inside. Tears of joy and grief may be experienced, and that I believe is normal.

I can recall in my first trimester with Champion-Jeral and Dominion knowing that I was pregnant before the test would even confirm it. What I have enjoyed most is sharing that joy with my husband, who usually calls that I am pregnant before I may even realize it. It is usually a hysterical moment I have that prompts him to say, "You may be pregnant."

I also serve as the lead project manager for our family business tasks, and I can attest to another level of focus that takes over when I am with child. There is a balance that business gives to the pregnancy process.

For anything to be birthed into life form proper nutrition, passion, and instinct must be applied. At this point, I am speaking to mom's who are more cautious to have children because they feel like they will miss their career.

You can have and be what you desire, do not miss your moment out of fear and critique from others.

Pregnancy is a journey that if relished in the moment I believe the mother can have a metaphysical experience. I have personally watched countless births online, and although I was not meeting anyone in person that could tell me a beautiful birth story, the information I sought after of other women giving birth, empowered me. Some births were longer or shorter, and many mothers can attest to realizing when they were ready for the child, that is when they were brought forth earth side.

I will share in the birth story of Champion how I delayed the actual birth process unknowingly and what I was doing to stall.

I have reasoned with myself that birth is a part of life, and

there is nothing to fear.

How do you get over your fears?

____

____

____

What are you most excited about when you think about

your birth?

____

____

____

At this moment, I would like for you to produce three

affirmations that you can recite as often as you can

remember to do so during your first trimester.

My birth affirmation

Date __/__/__

____

____

____

My birth affirmation

Date __/__/__

____

____

____

My birth affirmation

Date __/__/__

____

____

____

<u>Second Trimester</u>

I know what it is like to surrender to my body and the environment around me, while still dominating it at the same time. It is a quiet stillness, a shocking hum, and yet at the same time I have been blessed with the honor to have given birth to both of our sons at home. To some, it is extreme, but I have always been quite laissez-faire about many things, and again somehow, I dominate. Is that the recipe to success? Look, I do not know. I did not immediately notice this about my personality, but it became loud and clear when I became a parent. In order to dominate one must be prepared to surrender as the end result.

There is a quote from Sex and the City when Carrie Bradshaw says, "Everyone knows everything always works out as soon as you stop worrying about it."

Birth is mental and requires proper rest and nutrition, which in return feeds one's mind. Birth has taught me that society will not change until we change what is happening at birth.

If there is trauma in society, I am willing to bet there is trauma in the bloodline.

How do we produce a better society?

We must be willing to let new voices be heard to produce solutions based on first-hand experience accompanied with resources that will work.

<u>Symptoms:</u>

Vaginal Discharge

Increased Appetite

Increased Energy

Increased Intimacy

Slight Dizziness: Take Your Time

Skin Changes

Dental Changes

Slight Cramps

Belly Size Increase

Again, everyone is different and if embraced correctly by the mother I believe the resources that focus on the development of the baby can help you connect with the process. You must know what is happening inside of you to truly connect with your baby before they come earth-side. Recognize that they are growing and get more wrapped up in the miracle of life. Birth teaches you that there is a natural birthing process to life. Every day we open our eyes we receive another chance at life, which the hustle and bustle of life can make us take for granted.

My birth affirmation

Date __/__/__

____

____

____

My birth affirmation

Date __/__/__

____

____

____

My birth affirmation

Date __/__/__

____

____

____

<u>Third Semester</u>

This is the home stretch for you and your crowning moment is upon you. Realize that countless women have come before you and each of us had to be born to exist in life form. Allow that to sink in and connect with the power and strength that the after effect of birth will give to you.

While my God-sister was pregnant her husband announced, "That baby glow on you has you looking irresistible." It was the sweetest thing to hear, and she was blushing because he intentionally said it loud enough for other ears to hear.

Her hair was so thick and shiny, and that same day I complimented her as well. It was simply an effortless glow that being with child can produce. This is a true statement: there is a natural glory that only bringing forth life can give.

If you are ever looking at a woman and you cannot figure out her effervescence, it may be likely that she is a mother. She may be bubbly, happy, or just simply smitten by life because that is what the nurturing of children produces: Unexplainable Joy!

Birth requires a woman to be completely relaxed at her most intense and intimate state. How does one accomplish such a task? I believe she must have complete control over where and how she chooses to birth.

It can only be described as an individual experience that a mother must take full responsibility and accountability for—it is your life. For example, to the mothers who have had their children in the hospital or at a birth center with the support of a doula I am hearing in the community, it is a great match of teamwork. My husband has served as my doula for both births, and we find it better for us to have either a midwife present or in the case with our second son it was simply us.

Mothers who have chosen to do birth their way, are the women who must emerge to provide better solutions for society.

We must speak up and out for the voiceless group of women that are being mistreated and taken advantage of simply because they may live in poverty or are not empowered enough to make the best-informed decision on their pregnancy.

I do not believe abortion is the only way, as sometimes the fear and shock of motherhood has caused many to make decisions, they were not fully informed on making.

After reviewing the symptoms for the third trimester I will share both of my birth stories. The concluding section will be a list of resources that have empowered me.

<u>Symptoms</u>

Short or Long Sporadic Contractions

Shortness of Breath

Skin Stretching

Longer Naps

Eating Fuller Meals

Swelling of Feet: take it easy as best you can.

The final reminder is to take it easy as best you can. I encourage mothers to educate themselves to dispel the myth of fear in childbirth.

The gift of life was bestowed upon you, as the reader as well as me. When it is your time all you must do is own your experience, and I embrace the knowledge that only can be experienced when a mother owns her birth experience.

Unbeknownst to what others may think, there is no scorecard for judging another person. Everyone must win at what matters to them, by any means necessary.

My birth affirmation

Date __/__/__

____

____

____

My birth affirmation

Date __/__/__

____

____

____

My birth affirmation

Date __/__/__

____

____

____

Champion's Birth Story

Born: 1/23

Time: 3:16 AM

When my contractions began, I was lounging around, and I just finished having a sip of 100% grape juice. I enjoy the taste of grape juice or a sports electrolytes drink over anything else during each trimester. They quench my thirst, and the baby will always keep those two down. I later looked up the nutritional properties of grape juice and I saw that my body was craving a wonderful thing.

It makes sense that grape juice was also what set off that first tickle. The most hilarious mom instinct took place next; my phone rang. It was my mom checking on me, and I said I was fine. I was because it was not as if anything happened. I just felt a shift that was like a tickle from inside.

In real life, I could see our Young Champion being sincere enough to tickle me from inside to let me know he was ready to come out, something he enjoys doing to me now. His contractions felt like he was taking his fingers and moving them on the inside of me. Next, I got up and went to our lady's room and there I saw a mucus plug. I said to myself, "Ok, Ok."

What I should have done was acknowledge Champion alerting me that he was ready for us to begin the birth dance to bring him earth-side. For both of our son's as soon as I acknowledged them, they immediately came out. I do believe everything happens for a reason because I have learned something during both experiences.

The only expert I can ever believe there to be is a person who has walked the path through experience.

The birth process is the mother and baby figuring out the best way to get the process completed. I encourage mothers to connect with those first tickles and waves as they begin to roll from within. I wish that this were common sense, so after a **32**-hour experience I can share with you some things that may help you in whatever birth setting you are in.

1. I remained as calm as possible.
2. I notified my birth team: husband and midwife.
3. I paced myself.
4. I ate food, which subsided the waves and caused me to go to sleep during that 32-hour stretch.
5. I kept myself hydrated.

Back to the birth story: To describe our midwife, she is a Grand Midwife, which is the term used for seasoned midwives. At the time of our eldest birth, she was 71, and practicing for over 43 years.

Her brown dreadlocks stretched beyond her waist, and she kept a smirk on her face while monitoring me, and she and I knew my goal was to birth our first child at home instead of being in a hospital. When she arrived, she asked me to take walks and encouraged me to eat if I felt like it.

We walked to the market where my husband grabbed two sports drinks, (not energy drinks) and when we returned the Grand Midwife even got on our exercise bike.

Remember when I told you, I stalled my birth? Well, when I would sit on the exercise ball during waves that were intense, they would go away. I thought it was a good thing, and so at one point I even said to our Grand Midwife, "Is the yoga ball slowing down progress?" She said, "Maybe." I believe since I said it, it must have been true. I also remember frequently asking the waves and rushes to stop, and they would. Remember, the baby inside you can hear you and connect with you better than anyone else at this point. Try to use life giving affirmations to speak over the birth process.

The home birth experience can be categorized as a marathon or a sprint. It is such a unique experience that it is all its own. The woman needs as much nourishment as she desires during labor because there is no time frame on how short or long birth will be. While I was in labor with Champion, I was able to stomach the following:

Two Sports Drinks: I requested for one to be in the refrigerator and the other in the freezer. The first one I used during the first half of my contractions. From my personal experience, I can tell you for both of my births drinking a sports drink helped me get those electrolytes in. I do believe light sips can be refreshing during the birthing process. Right at transition, I was hot and cold at the exact same time. My husband passed me the sports drink that was half frozen and it was the best thing in that moment because I needed something to get me through that final moment.

Spaghetti w/Bread: This is the first meal I ate, and our Grand Midwife shared in the dinner. My husband was preparing the food during the process. I am eternally grateful for our connection and understanding. He is what I consider to be my doula, and no one has advocated better for me than him. After I ate, I can recall the contractions subsiding and I was able to take a nap.

Chicken w/Mashed Potatoes and Corn: I know, and it was so delicious! To this day, I told my husband that was a very tasty treat because I did not eat much. I can recall the flavor and the crunch being just a reminder that I was in a race, and I just needed to remain nourished. There are some marathon runners that can eat a banana or orange in the middle of a race simply to keep up their stamina. I also took a nap after each meal, which helped. The first birth, I simply just didn't know what to expect so I eventually surrendered, and I believe that is what birth is all about: complete surrender to the process.

In the defense of many hospitals, I could see there being a level of difficulty to provide all women with a certain level of care. I do believe everyone should always try to do the absolute best for mother, baby, and the overall family. I was nibbling on comfort food that was being made with love and focus. Again, my husband has realized the best thing to do for me in birth is just to be there for me the best way possible. I desire more couples to share that experience.

I was in labor with our first-born son for 32 hours, as far as when the contractions began until the birth. Active pushing, I would say was about 1 hour because I was holding my breath to push. It is incorrect to do that because a mother needs to breathe more than anything in between the rushes.

 I was risking passing out and our Grand Midwife said, "Ok, bare down like you have to go to the bathroom." I simply said, "Ok" and that moment registered with my brain. Then suddenly, she says, "STOP! Stop pushing."

I was laying on my back, which in hindsight was not the best position to bring forth the baby because I felt like I was hunched over constricting the passageway. My intuition was correct and with my husband and midwife in between my legs I heard her calmly say, "The cord is around the neck, and we need to push him in and then shimmy the cord around the body." Again, I said "Ok" because there was nothing else, I could do, and just trust what she was saying. So, my husband held the baby and there was a very quick push in and then he was out.

We kept the gender a surprise, and so it was a sure delight to hear my husband say, "It's a boy. It's Champion." I can attest to not even resonating with the crashing of the waves I felt as Champion was ready to come forth. I was in complete amazement that I did it! We did it, as a family.

I was encouraged to partake in eating while going through my contractions, that was truly the reason I was successfully able to have a first-time home birth. I was nourished and hydrated, and then I would rest. It was a rhythm that one cannot explain only experienced with a support team that understands the mother's vision.

By the time I brought forth Champion and I checked my email about fifteen mothers from the UK (Tellmeagoodbirthstory.com) sent me messages of encouragement. If there is one thing, I can say about the home birthing community is that it is extremely inclusive.

The love and encouragement from the mothers are what has encouraged me to author this book.

Note: This book is not to promote home birth as the only option for bringing forth one's child. Home birth is something that if a mother is motivated by her own convictions and she is healthy, she can do it, consecutively. I also see the value in hospitals, and as a society we just all must work together towards better birth outcomes.

Dominion's Birth Story

Born: 12/14

Time: 4:33 A.M.

For the purpose of connection, I will be going more line by line on the topic of Dominion's birth, which was 6 hours.

These were the following things I did differently:

1. I rested for as long as possible even during contractions, and when they intensified, I embraced the fact that the best thing I could do is push.

2. I looked myself in the mirror right before the birth waves went roaring and simply said aloud, "I can do this. We can do this."

3. I placed a scarf over the door and used it to steady myself and push, which then prompted my water to burst.

4. I nibbled on food and managed to eat a big meal that day simply to get those nutrients in before the race began. I was not interested in food once it ramped up.

5. I had two sports drinks that I sipped simply to curb dehydration (I am not a DR; it is just what worked for me).

6. I let my husband sleep until I knew that the rushes were too intense for me to manage by my own mental strength.

7. The birth was unassisted with a midwife friend on the phone to help guide my husband.

8. I transferred to the hospital afterwards and when the doctor asked to check my vagina with his two fingers I said, "No, thank you. I did not tear." He then picked up a flashlight and said, "There are no lacerations." Surprisingly, he could find out the

same information without sticking his fingers

anywhere close to me. At the same time, my

husband and son were coming in so I am grateful

for my instincts because I also know my husband

would not have allowed me to be touched in such a

way.

<u>Resources</u>

All a mother must do is begin the research for birth. Begin with reading books and look at the reviews before you buy them. You are looking for confident mothers that express how the information helped them in their journey. The fact of birth is that the person who has the most intimate and close experience is the woman carrying the actual child inside of her. As many of us invest in our education to obtain higher knowledge the same must be done for the mother, if she genuinely wants to get over any fear of childbirth.

The mother should educate herself on what is going on during the natural birthing process, and it will take the sting out of birth. Many mothers forget the birth as soon as they bring them for earth-side in a positive environment.

You can remove fear through information if you consume enough of it to change your mental perspective. For example, I was afraid of snakes until I found out if you cut off their head they will die. I researched it and even watched it a few times online and so when people say they are afraid of snakes I always announce, "We'll just have to slice that head clean off."

Fear should not exist when research is present:

1. How to Raise A Healthy Child In Spite of Your Doctor by Dr. Joseph Murphy
2. Freebirth by Sarah Schmid
3. Active Birth by Janet Balaskas
4. Birth Without Fear by January Harshes
5. Mama Says Home Birth by Miquilaue Young
6. Spontaneous Joyful Natural Birth by Natasha Panzer
7. Ina May's Guide to Childbirth by Ina May Gaskin
8. Orgasmic Birth by Elizabeth Davis
9. Birthing from Within by Pam England and Rob Horowitz
10. Childbirth Without Fear by Grantly Dick-Read
11. The Thinking Woman's Guide to a Better Birth by Henci Goer
12. Babies Are Not Pizzas: They're Born Not Delivered by Rebecca Dekker
13. Supernatural Childbirth by Jackie Mize
14. Placenta- The Forgotten Chakra by Robin Lim
15. The Complete Book of Pregnancy and Childbirth by Sheila Kitzinger
16. The Essential Homebirth Guide by Jane E. Dritcha
17. The Baby Book by James Sears MD.
18. The Business of Being Born by Ricki Lake
19. Orgasmic Birth the Documentary by Debra Pascali-Bonaro
20. The Ultimate Guide to Sex After Baby: Secrets to Love and Intimacy by Debra Pascali-Bonaro

Additional Resources

Online Resources

http://www.tellmeagoodbirthstory.com/

https://www.freebirthsociety.com/

https://thepositivebirthcompany.co.uk/blog

https://www.unassistedchildbirth.com/

Baby Midwives Blog

https://blog.feedspot.com/birth_blogs/

https://www.verywellfamily.com/birth-videos-about-natural-childbirth-2758298

Movies

https://theempoweredmama.com/birth-documentaries-that-will-blow-your-mind/

A Positive Home Birth Video

https://youtu.be/oKfpJ-upxfk

Social influencers

https://www.parents.com/parenting/money/family-finances/6-instagram-influencer-moms-spill-their-secrets/

Breastfeeding
&

Empowered

Elizabeth Clyde

To Be Continued...

If this book helped you, I would love

to connect with you. Please email me

at biz@elizabethclyde.com.

Truly best wishes to you and may

you find JOY in the JOURNEY!

Mrs. Elizabeth Clyde

Clyde-Family.com

www.ingramcontent.com/pod-product-compliance
Lightning Source LLC
Chambersburg PA
CBHW031427250726
48656CB00002B/875